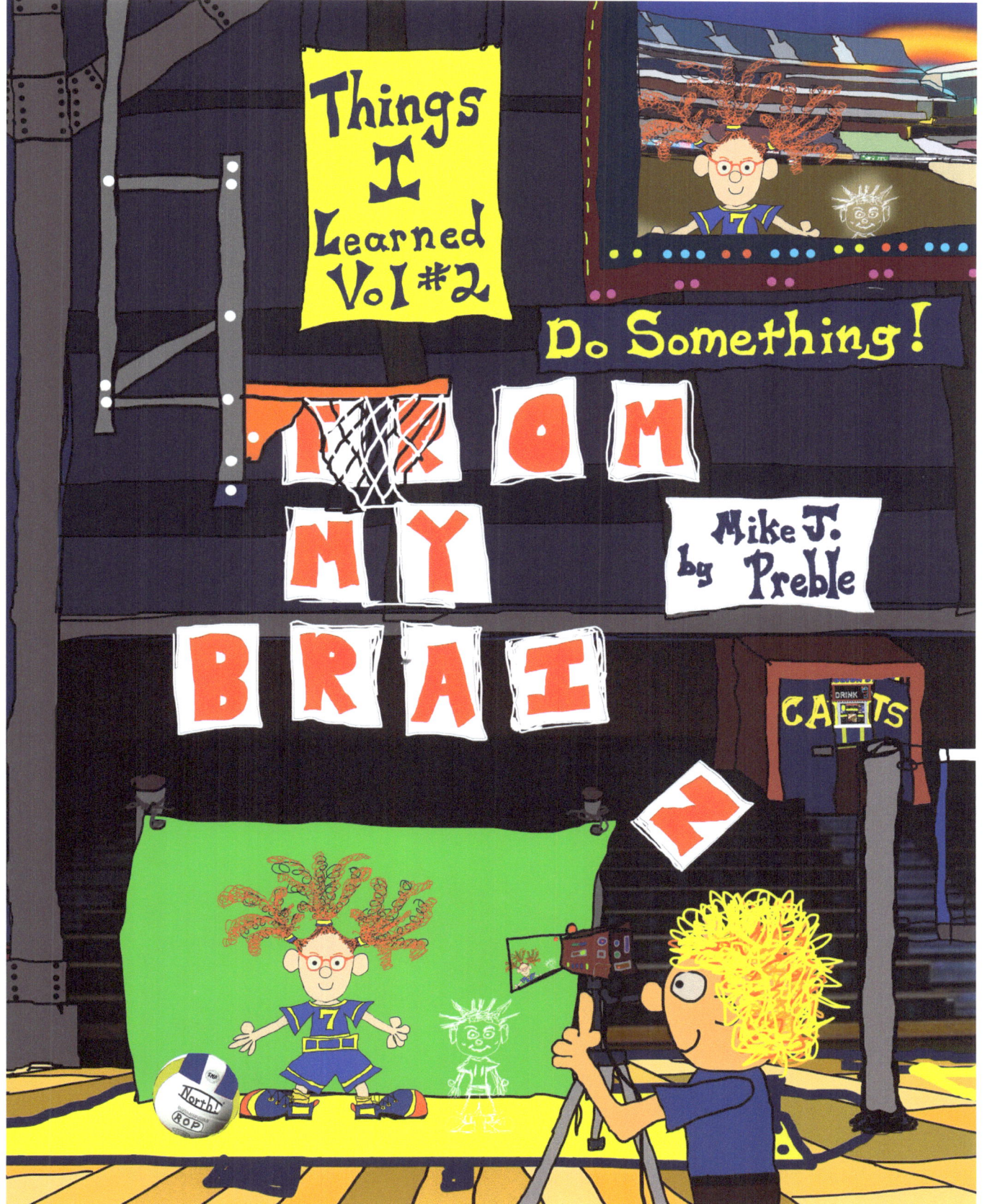

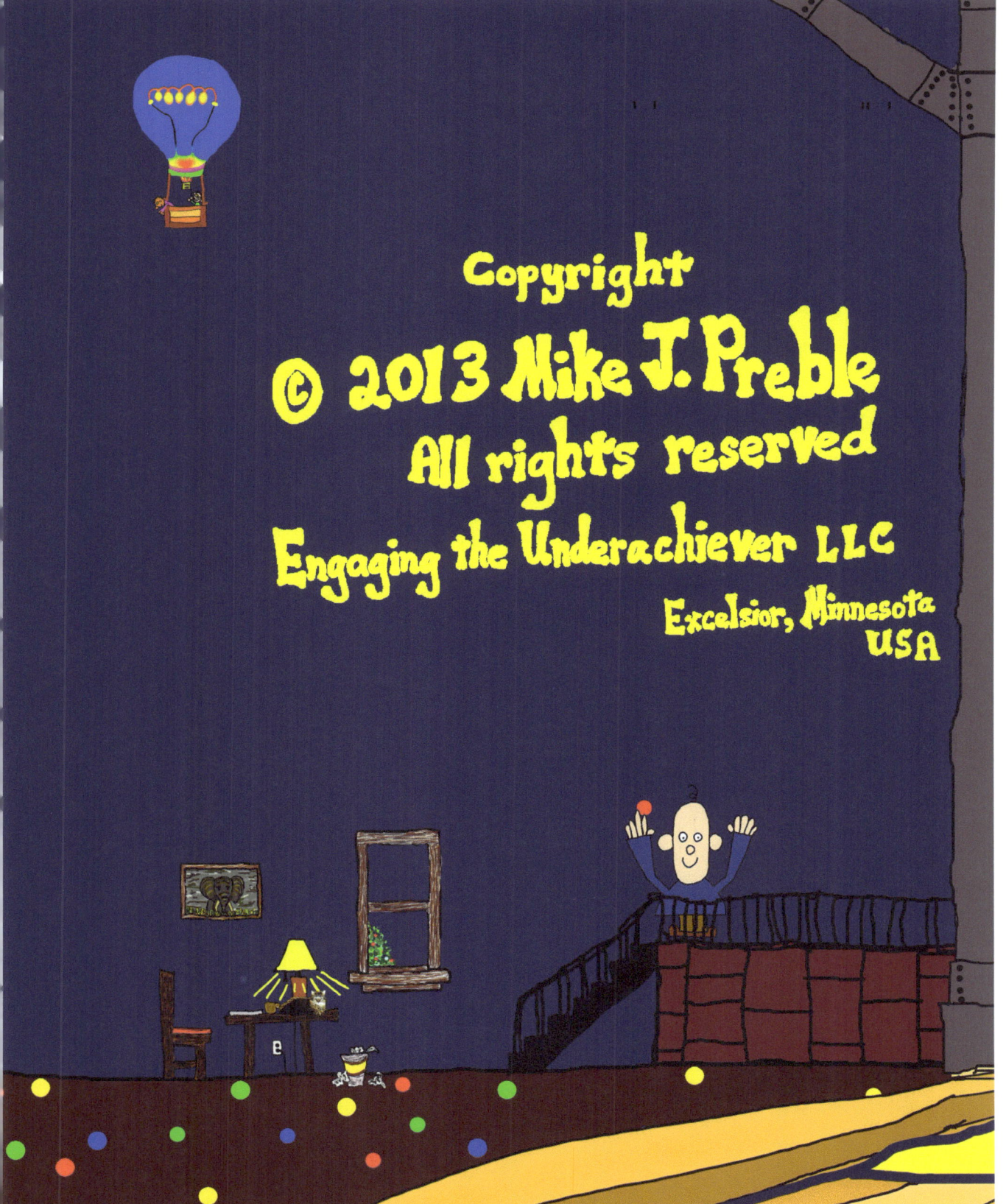

Dedicated to
the Real
Angie Ropp
and
"Oh, Snap!"

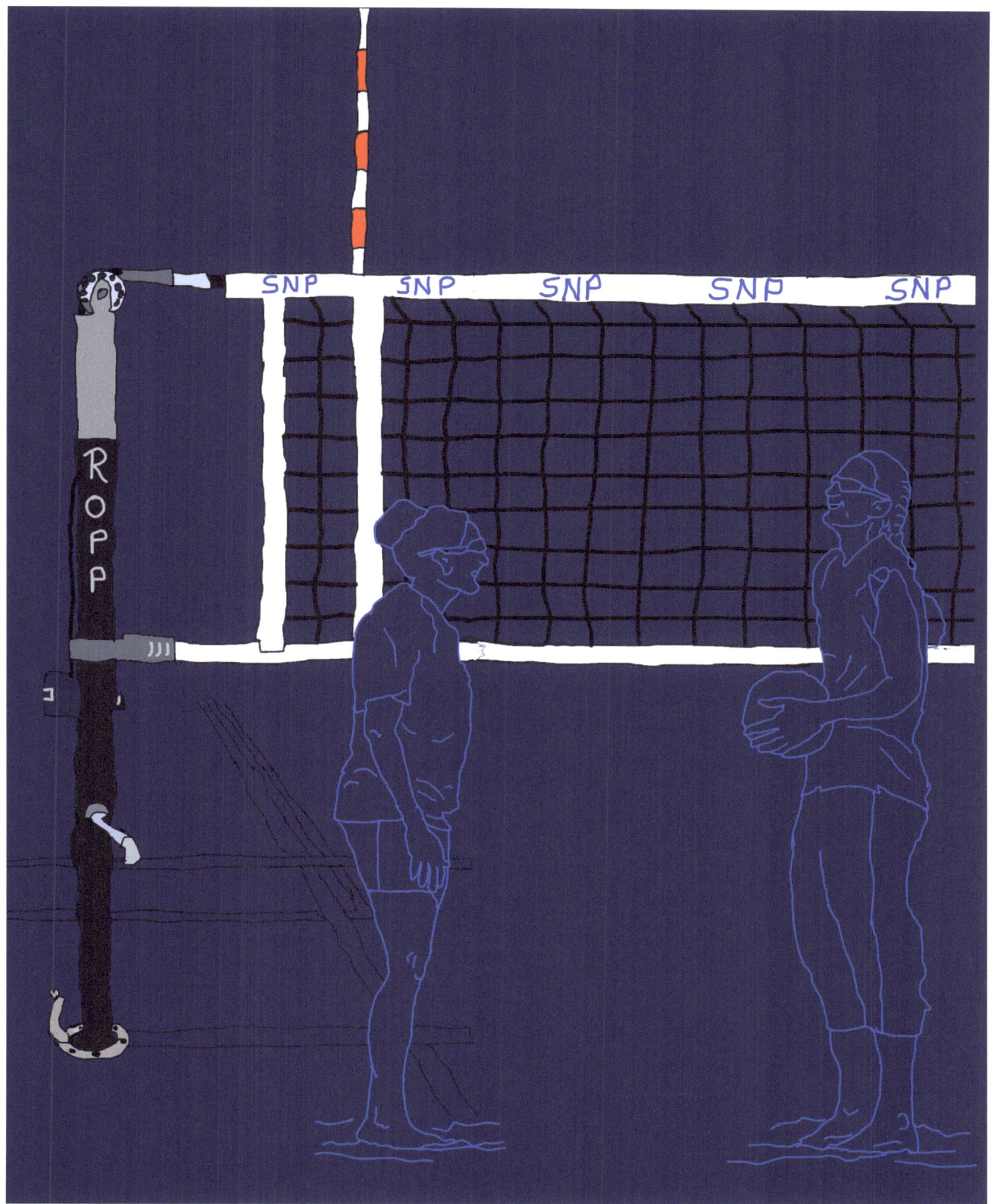

Table of Contents

Do Something! .... P.   1

What-cha Gonna Do? .... p.   7

Some Planning (Required) .... p.   13

CCoQ&A .... p.   21

Do Something!

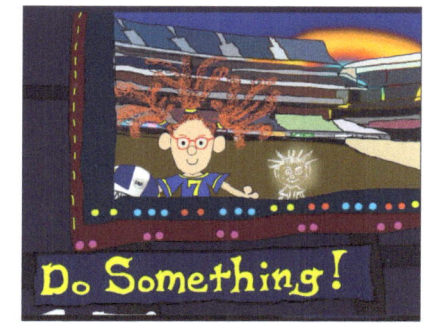

Howdy, everyone. My name is Angie Ropp and you're watching "Do Something!" The show where we say, "Do Something!"

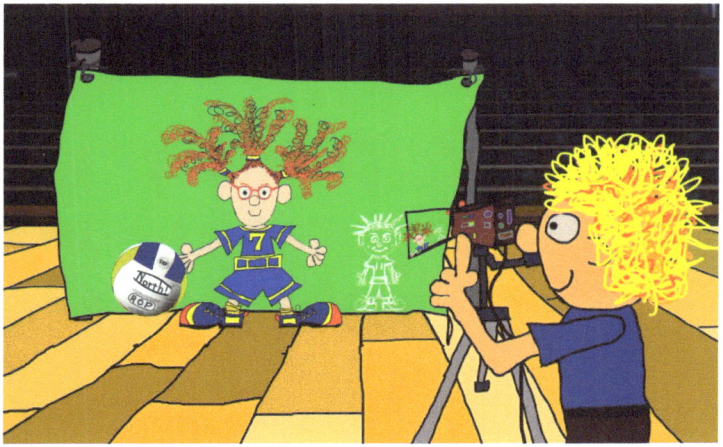

As you can see, it's a beautiful spring day at this magnificent outdoor stadium (actually, it's a Saturday afternoon in January and we're in my school gym, but, hey, thanks to Goulasche Press behind the camera and Green Screen magic, we can be anywhere we want to be.

We could be climbing a mountain, sailing the ocean, or flying a space ship to the moon, or…,)

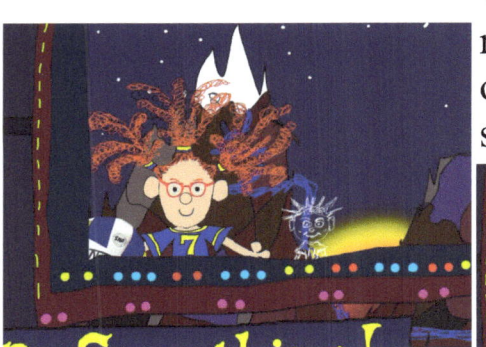

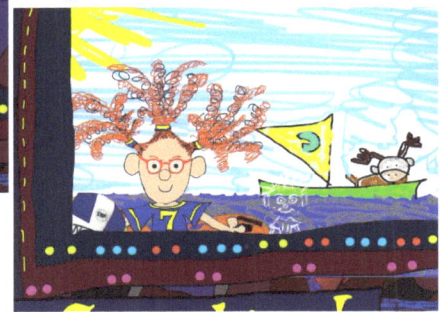

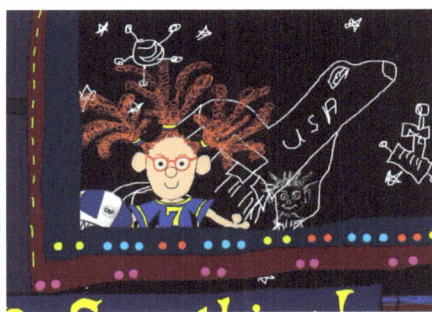

What? Oh, right. Or we could start here, where we are and just "Do Something!"

Today, we are going to show you how to get in shape, what it takes to be in shape and then, what you need to do, every day, to stay in shape.

We're talking about physical shape (your body's muscle tone and weight) and mental shape (the thinking and learning processes in your brain.)

1

Standing next to me is my partner, and my best friend, who is about to -- "Oh, Snap!"…, where are you going?

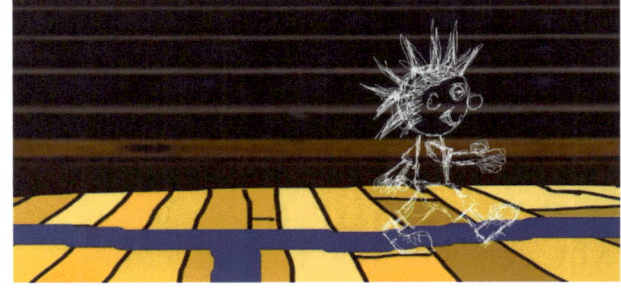

Well, Ladies and Gentlemen, Boys and Girls, it appears "Oh, Snap!" is going for a walk, along the edge of the gym floor, all the way to the corner.

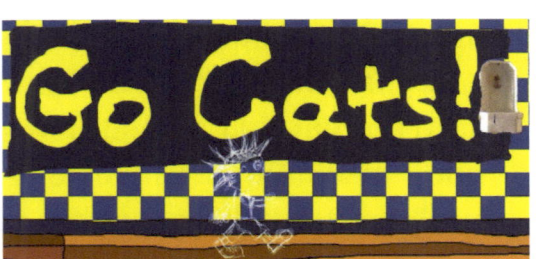

Now she's turning the corner, and walking along the back wall. It looks like, yes, she's going all-the-way-around the entire gym floor, walking in a very steady, measured fashion.

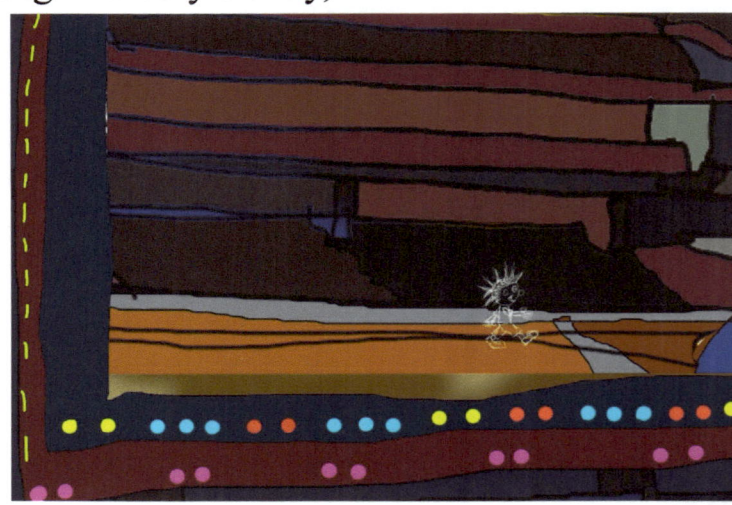

Take a look at the Jumble-Screen high up in the rafters. You can see her walking way out in what is normally left field, but is now covered with a special sand mixture for the North American Outdoor Beach Volleyball Tournament, coming up next, in most areas, except for the West Coast. So, check your local listings.

Oh, and I'd like to say we're also streaming live, over the internet, at: www.AngieRoppOhSnap.com.

(What? No streaming? Oh, okay. Sorry.)

I guess we're not streaming right now. But after the show you'll be able to go online and check out video clips posted by…, (What? No video clips right after the show? You're going to visit your grandparents in Duluth? And you won't be back until tomorrow night. Okay, then.)

I guess the video clips will be posted as soon as Goulasche gets back from visiting his Grandparents in Duluth.

Oh, well. As they say, "The Show Must Go On."

Hello, everyone, my name is Angie Ropp and this is "Do Something!" The show where we show you how to get in shape, how to be in shape and how to stay in shape, and, as an added bonus, how to improve your brain - your thinking skills, your memory skills, as well as your imagination and creativity.

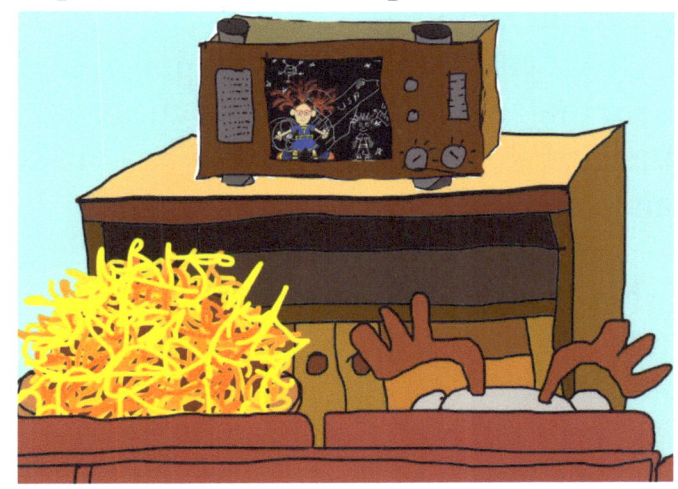

So, sit back and relax, and let us do all the work. (Why should you have to do all the work? Think about it.)

Is everyone ready? Comfy? Feet up and relaxed? Something to munch on? A nice, soft pillow? Well, then. Let's get started.

First of all, the most important thing to keep in mind is…,
Well, okay then. I guess "Oh, Snap!" has rounded the last corner and is just about back from her trip all the way around the gym floor.

Did you have a nice walk?
128? Oh, that's how many steps it was.
One minute, 37 seconds? That's how long it took you.

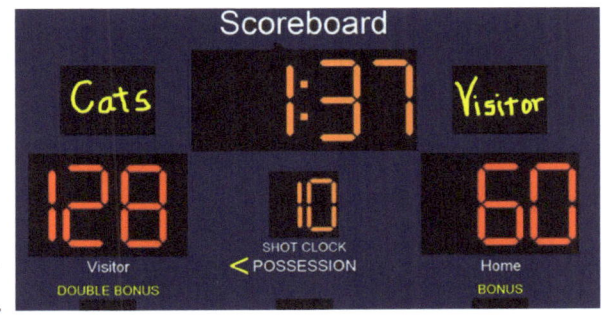

And now it looks like you are standing on one leg, balancing, while counting to twenty. Very nice.

Now for the other leg, standing, counting, backwards, from twenty.

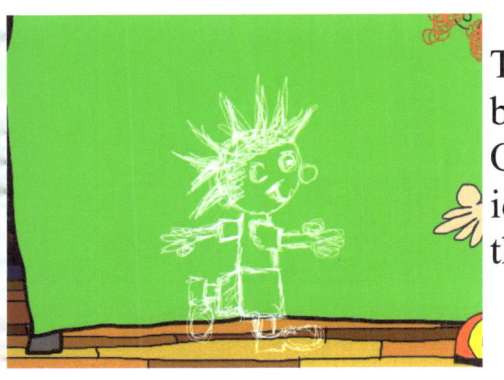

That's excellent balancing, with both sides of the body given equal treatment.
Oh, you say you practice it? That's a very good idea. Everyone knows the things you practice are the things you get better at and remember.

Now you are hopping and counting, at the same time.

Hopping and counting by 2s.

That's a new idea. Counting by 2s to 20 while hopping.

Now you're skipping. Skipping while counting. Counting by 3s. I guess since they call it 'Skip-Counting' why not skip and count. All the way up to 30.

Leaping! Wow! Those are giant leaps while you're counting by 4s on each leap. Counting by 4s all the way to 40. Amazing.

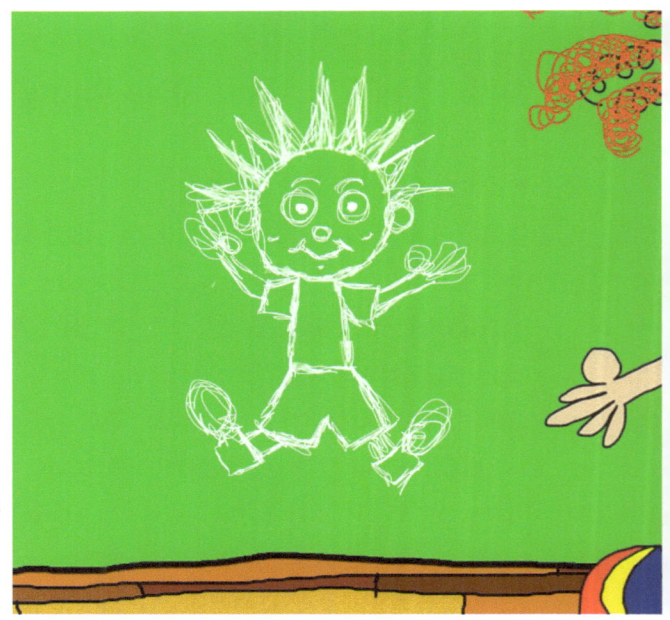

Don't tell me: Counting by 5s? While doing Jumping Jacks. That takes both coordination and rhythm. Might I ask how you do on your times tables?

You know all of the 2s, 3s, 4s, and 5s. Well, is there any wonder? You're moving about, balancing and counting, hopping, leaping and jumping while skip-counting. You are working your body and your brain, both at the same time. That's what this program is all about.

You are definitely a "Do Something!" action girl.

Well, there you have it. "Do Something!", and "Oh, Snap!" has just shown us how.

That concludes our first lesson and our first show.

We hope you enjoyed it. Let us know what you think by sending us an email.

Don't forget to check out our website to see all the cool things Goulasche will be putting up there in the very near future.

Good bye. Thanks for watching.

See you next time.

And don't forget: "Do Something!"

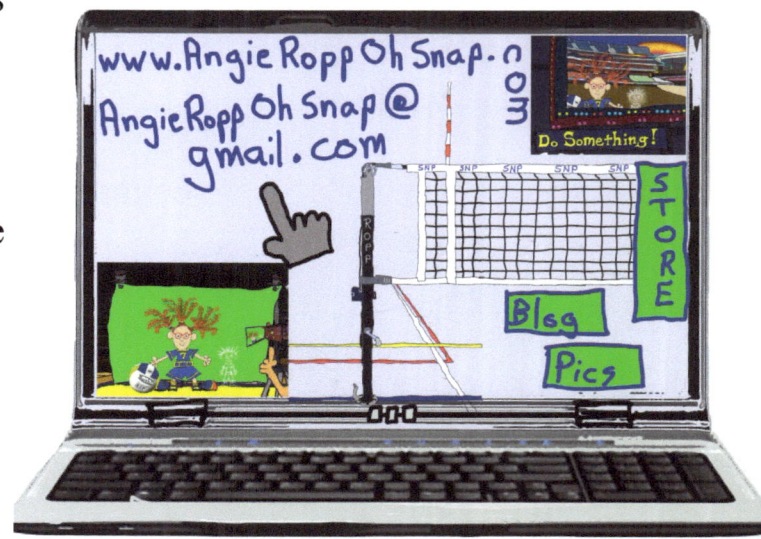

(Wow. That was great. Thanks, Goulasche.
"Oh, Snap!" You're a genius. You have such excellent ideas.
Goulasche, "Oh, Snap!" and I can take down the green screen and roll it up, if you like.
Do you need any help with those cords?
Maybe we can help carry everything out to the car.
Is your mom or dad picking you up?
My mom's in the hallway, by the concession stand. She had to do a few things to get ready for next Saturday's game. Are you going? I'm going.
"Oh, Snap!", you're going, aren't you?
We can pick you up about 5 PM, if you like. Maybe stop for burgers.)

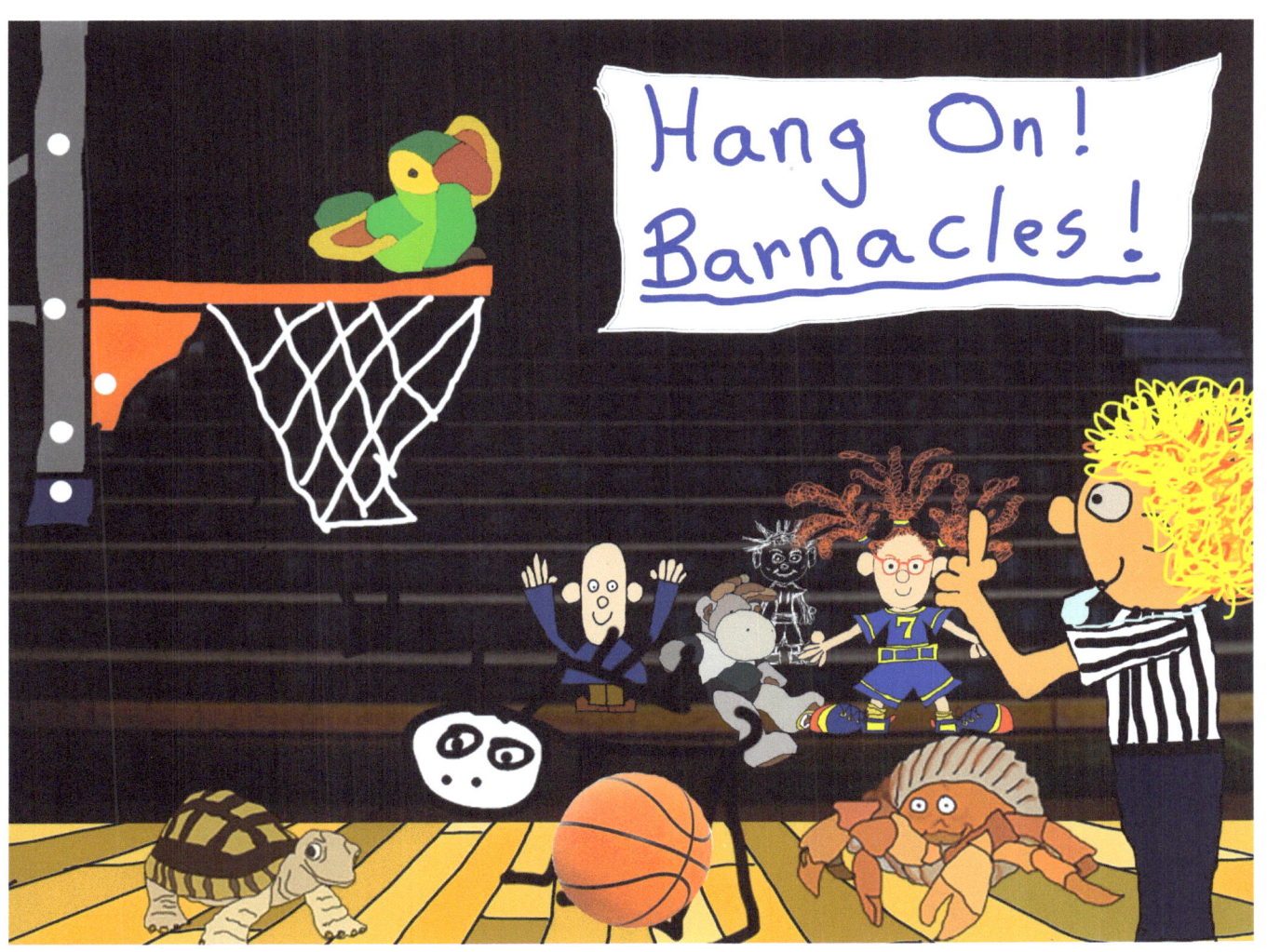

WHAT-CHA GONNA DO

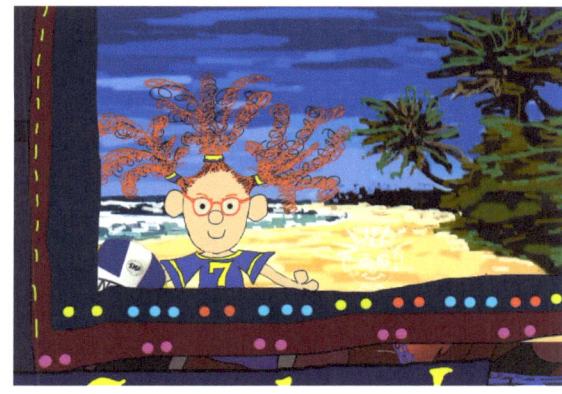

Well, howdy, everyone.

Glad to see you're back for more action.

You're watching "Do Something!" The show where we say "Do something!"

Today, we are going to answer that age-old question that nearly everyone asks and is seldom answered: "What-cha gonna do?"

You may have noticed we are broadcasting, live, from somewhere near the ocean. Actually, we're on a sunny beach in beautiful Hawaii (not really) and that's the magnificent Pacific ocean right behind us (no, it's not.)

"Oh, Snap!" and I are here to show you a variety of ideas and activities that could easily be used to answer that question everyone asks, especially when you are bored and can't think of anything creative or fun or interesting to do.

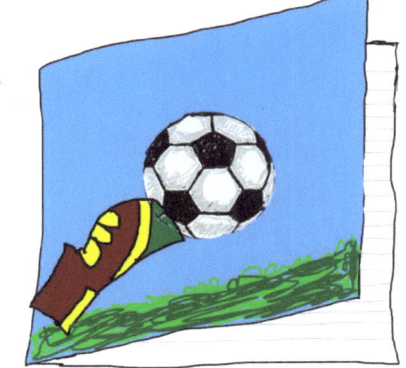

As you can see, sort of, "Oh, Snap!" has a…, Well, what do you have?

It looks like a box. A shoe box, with a hole in the lid. A hole with a flap. And the flap covers a hole that just fits your hand.

She's reaching inside the box and pulling out something.

It looks like…, yes, it is a card. Is that a card? It's a card.

A 3 x 5 notecard and it is folded, in half - like a tiny book. It's a 3 x 5 Note Card Activity Book.

And what is the 3 x 5 Note Card Activity Book for?

Oh, it's for this next activity. Well, that's sweet.

So, is there something written inside the note card?

Yes? Many things? Okay.

It has a picture on the front. A soccer ball and a foot.

Is that your foot?

So, this card has things to do with a soccer ball and your foot. Is that right?

7

Good. And now what? Open the card?

A list: "5 things to do with a soccer ball and your foot." And…

You want me to read them out loud and you'll demonstrate? Super.

Ladies and Gentlemen, Boys and Girls, "Oh, Snap!" and her 3x5 Notecard Activity Book: "5 things to do with a soccer ball and your foot."

Ready? Set! Demonstrate...

#1. Kick the ball, with one foot, for one minute. Okay, let's see it.

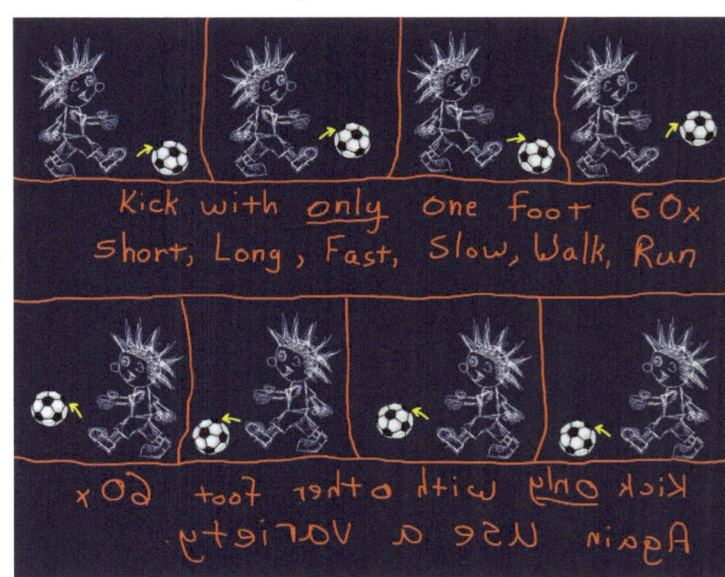

Wow! Look at that, kicking the ball with only one foot all around the yard.

How do you know one minute is up?

You count to yourself.

What do you count?

You count the kicks?

I see. That's how you get to 60. What if someone can't count to 60?

Count to 10, and then count to ten, again. Do that 6 times in a row. That makes 60. Super.

What do you do when you are finished? Do it, again, with the other foot. Super. And then, after that? Take turns?

Left-right, left-right. That's taking one idea and making it into 3 activities.

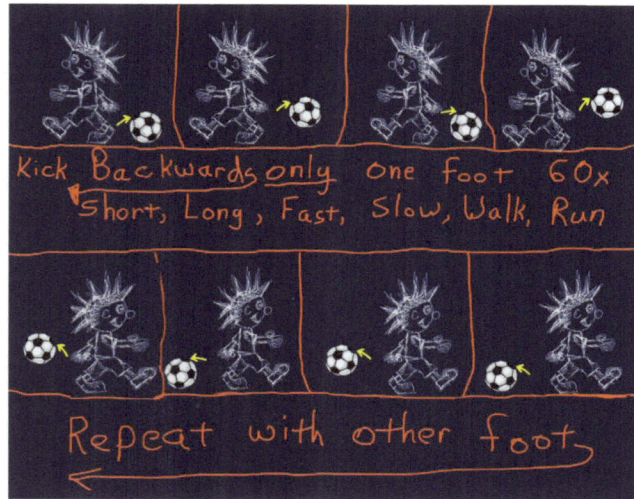

Now for the second one.

#2. Kick the ball backwards, same as #1.

That would be using your heal? Okay, and then, like in #1, you use only one foot and count to 60. Then the other and count to 60, and then switch between each foot for a third count of 60? Great.

#3 says "Footsie Catch." What does "footsie catch" mean?

Bounce the ball off your foot. Must take a lot of practice and concentration.

How many times? 60, again? Okay.

What happens if you miss?

Just keep counting to 60. Good.

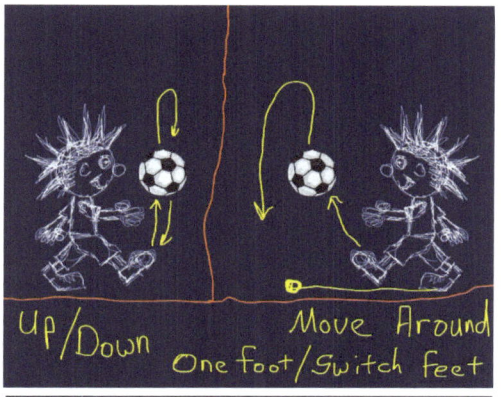

Now, #4: "Foot-Foot Stop" What's that?

Oh, you pass the ball from one foot to the other while moving about, forward, backwards and sideways, and then you stop. And spin around, start-and-stop. That's a lot of maneuvering.

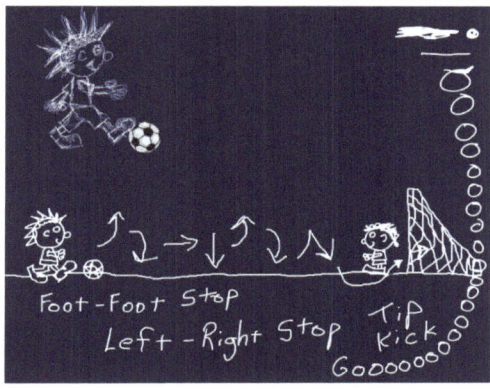

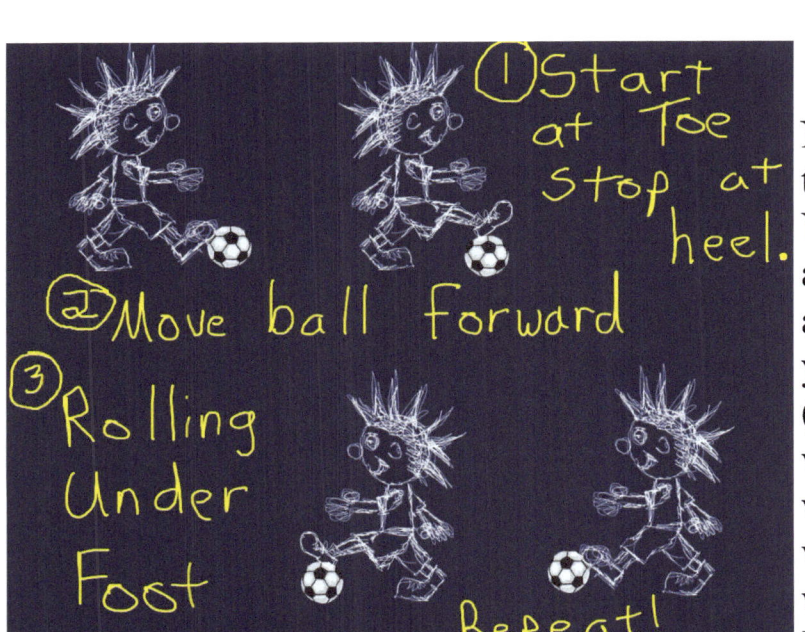

Now, #5: "Foot Roll" Well, that needs some demonstration. You have two cones set up, about…, how far apart? 10 giant steps. Okay, and then, you're going to push the ball (not kick it, but push the ball) with your toe, and then stop it with your heal. And then push with the other foot and stop it with your heal.

It's kind of like rolling the ball along, not really trying to get anywhere real fast. Is that the goal? Good.

And when you get to the cone you turn around. Let me guess, do this ten times?

Wow. That's an amazing list of things to do with a soccer ball and your foot. What other kinds of cards do you have in your shoe box?

9

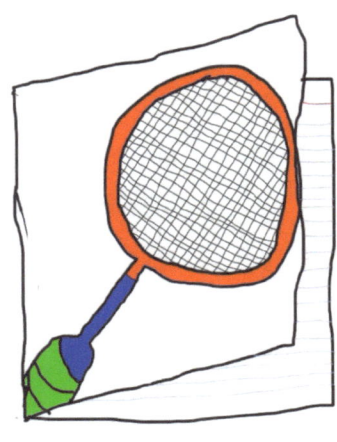

"5 Things to do with a badminton racket and a birdie."
That looks interesting.

"Skateboarding Fun."
Skateboarding really makes you work on your balance and endurance.

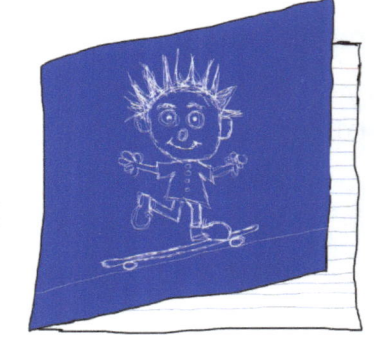

"Rope-Skipping Games"
I love rope skipping, but I was never good at "Red-Hot-Peppers."

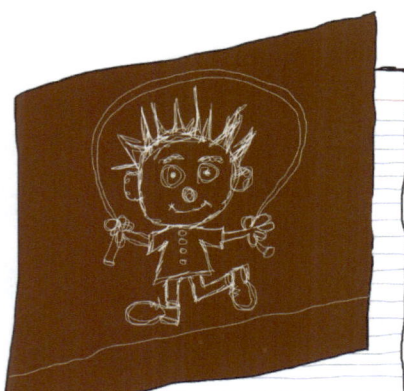

"Baseball Catch and Other Games"
Catch is a great game for developing Hand-Eye coordination, which is also practicing your reading skills.

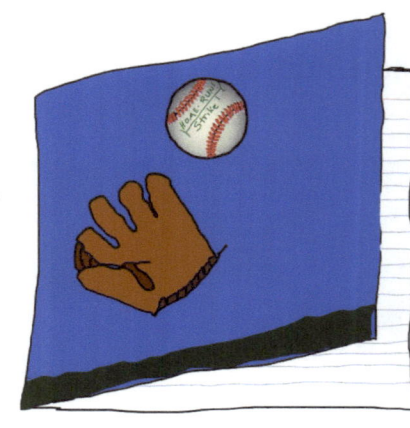

"Roller Blading Around the Block"
Good, you have on your knee pads, elbow and wrist pads and a helmet. You should always think of safety when you are playing.

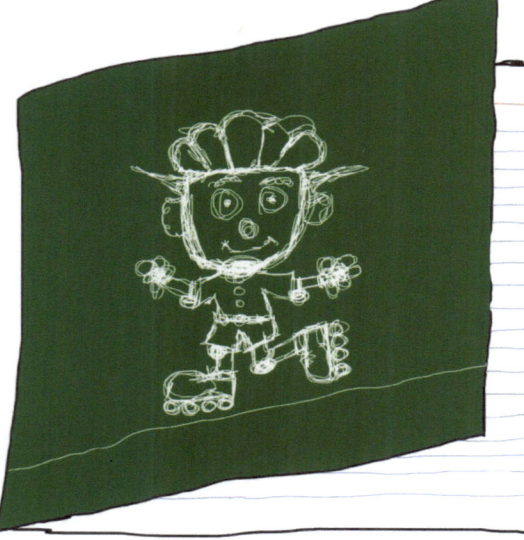

"Biking"
Riding a bike is a super workout for your large muscles, balance control, endurance, heart and lungs… It's one of the best things you can do. Just make sure you watch for other cars and obey all traffic rules.

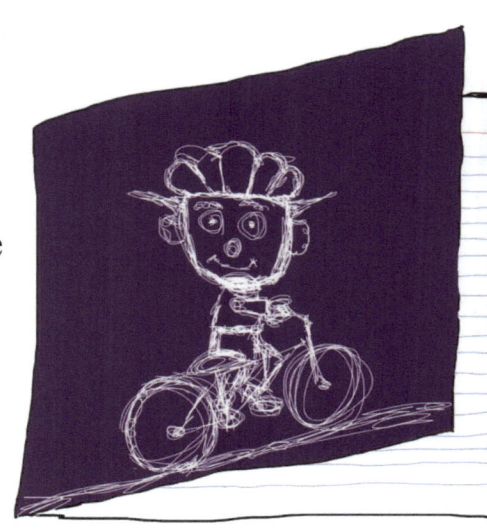

That is a super creation and collection of activities for moving about.

And I suppose you could do these alone or with some friends.

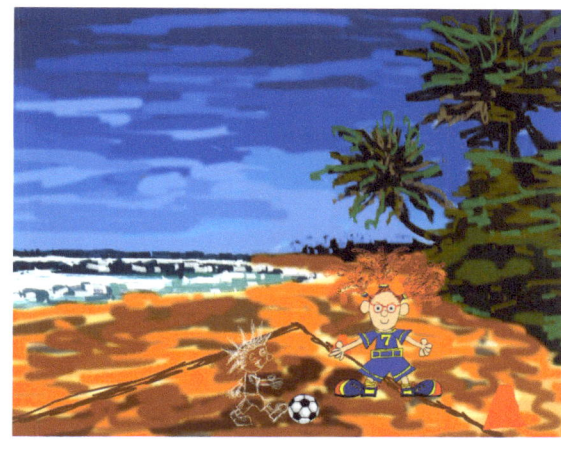

Well, thank you, everyone, for tuning in.

We'll post the other activities on our website.

Good bye for now, and have a nice and active day.

(Wow, that was a great show. Thank you "Oh, Snap!" Thank you, Goulasche.

Email? No, I haven't checked that, yet.

Next show? "Oh, Snap!" and I were thinking about showing how to make a plan of action, for exercising and nutrition. You know, like a daily schedule, or a weekly chart. Maybe keep a journal.

I'll email you some ideas. Thanks.)

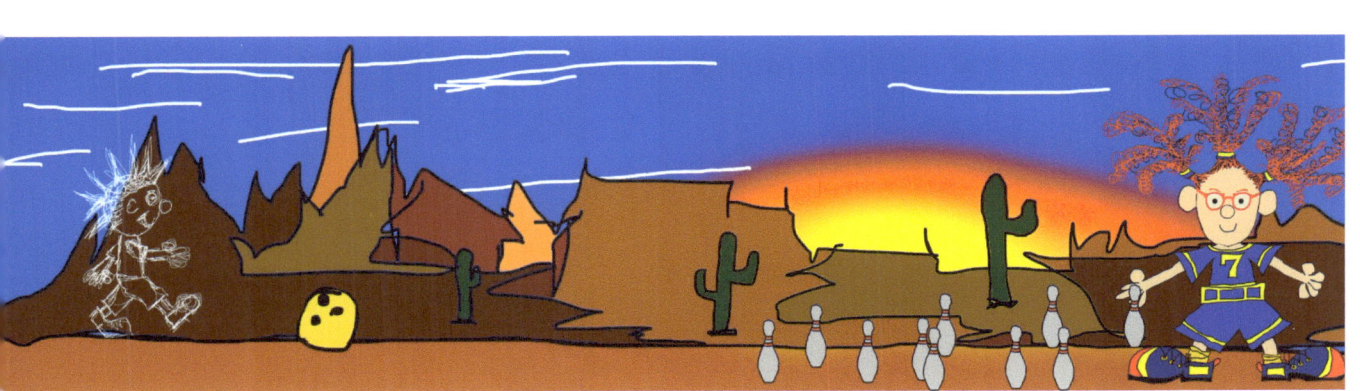

Some Planning
(required)

Howdy, everyone.

My name is Angie Ropp, and standing next to me is my partner, "Oh, Snap!" Goulasche Press is behind the camera, and this is "Do Something!" The show where we say "Do something!" and then we show you something to do.

Today, we are going to…,

Yes?

Oh, right.   Thank you. I forgot.

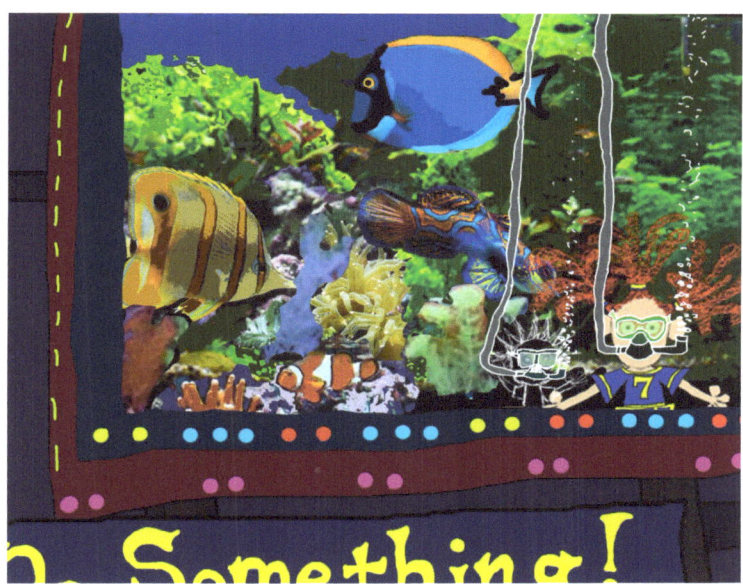

Ladies and Gentlemen, Boys and Girls, "Oh, Snap!" just reminded me to tell you where we are, today.

We are broadcasting, live, from under water, in the super fantastic "Aquarium Classroom of Tomorrow" - AqCOT Hall, located on the rolling hill just off Lilac Lane, not far from downtown Chicago, to talk to you about today's installment of "Do Something!" that we are calling "Some Planning (required)."

In today's show we'll explain how to make your own plans for activities; A Plan for physical health and endurance, A Plan for improving muscular strength and flexibility, A Plan for maintaining proper diet and nutrition, A Plan for active learning and problem solving skills development and A Plan for personal goal setting, achievement and success.

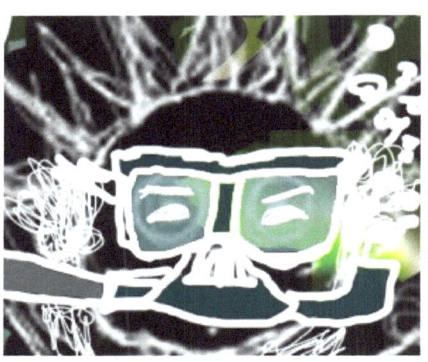

"Oh, Snap!" why are you covering your ears and squinting your eyes?

It sounds like a lot of work, but it's not, once you understand what to do and how to make it happen.

13

As everyone knows, it's very easy to do nothing. All you have to do to do nothing is -- do nothing. It's even easier to keep on doing nothing, because you have plenty of practice to get good at it.

It is very difficult to be active. It is even more difficult to stay active.

Try running and jumping and throwing and catching and practicing and playing all day long. It is tiring! Especially at first, if you haven't been doing much of anything for quite a while.

Your body is out of shape and out of practice. But, after a while, it becomes easier, and it keeps on getting easier, the more you practice. Plus, the benefits are enormous.

"Oh, Snap!" Where are you going?

She's walking way over to the other side of the gym. Now she's pushing a white board back. Oooooh! Oil those wheels.

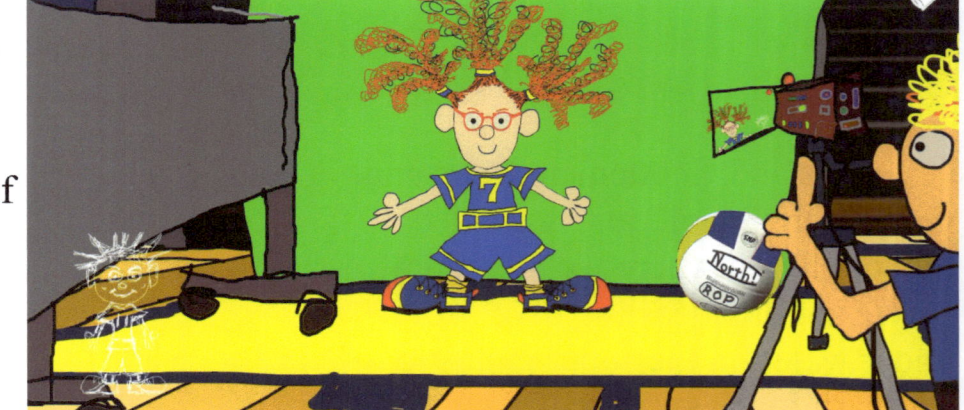

"Oh, Snap!" What are you going to do with a white board?
Draw? Draw what?
Pictures? Charts and graphs? Activities? Actions?
That sounds…, interesting.
You're going to draw while I'll speak? Like a magic "show and tell".
Goulasche, I guess you will have to switch the camera back-and-forth, a lot.

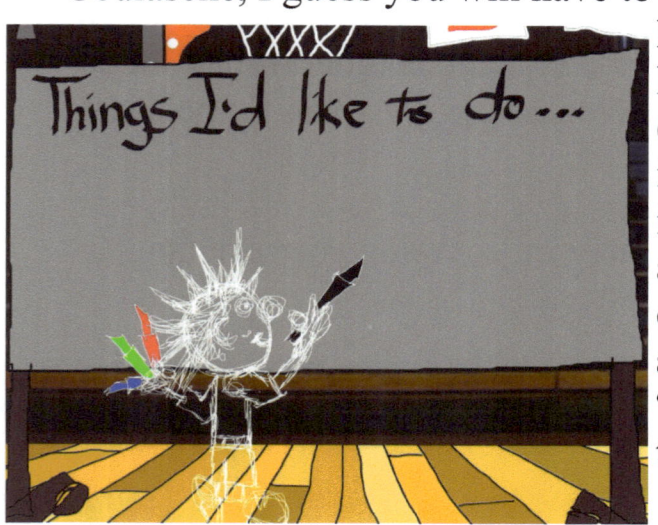

Here we go:
In making a plan, the first thing to do (well, it doesn't have to be the first thing) is make a list: Think of it as gathering ingredients, like getting pots and pans and food for cooking or paper and crayons, scissors and markers and glue for an art project. Once you have a pile of "ingredients" it's easier to to make something.

14

First of all, let's list some goals:

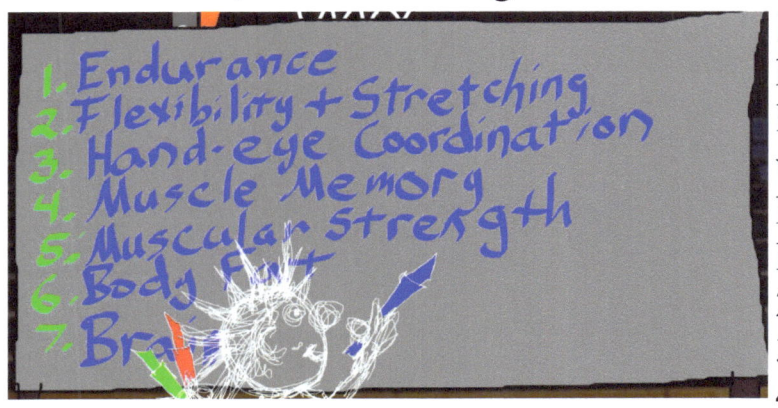

1. Endurance. What? You don't know what endurance is?
It means "to be able to keep going when you're doing something." How to spell it?"
E - N - D - U - R - A - N - C - E.
2. Flexibility and stretching
3. Hand-eye coordination
4. Muscle memory
5. Muscular strength
6. Body Fat
7. Improved brain functioning: Thinking skills, imagination, creativity, memory, problem solving, planning, communication, coordination, production.

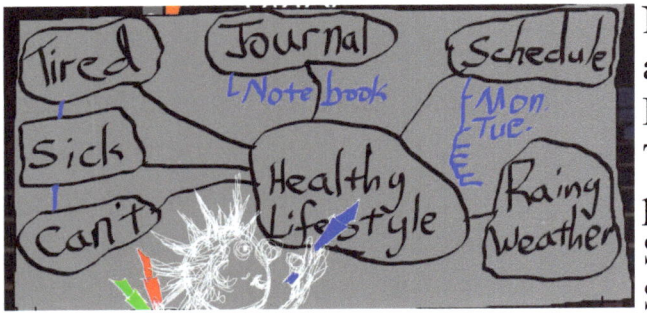

Now, another way to get ideas is to make a web, something like a spider's web. Put Healthy Lifestyle in the center circle. Then put some lines going out. Now, let's put some words on those lines: Schedule, Journal, Rainy Weather, Tired, Sick, Can't.

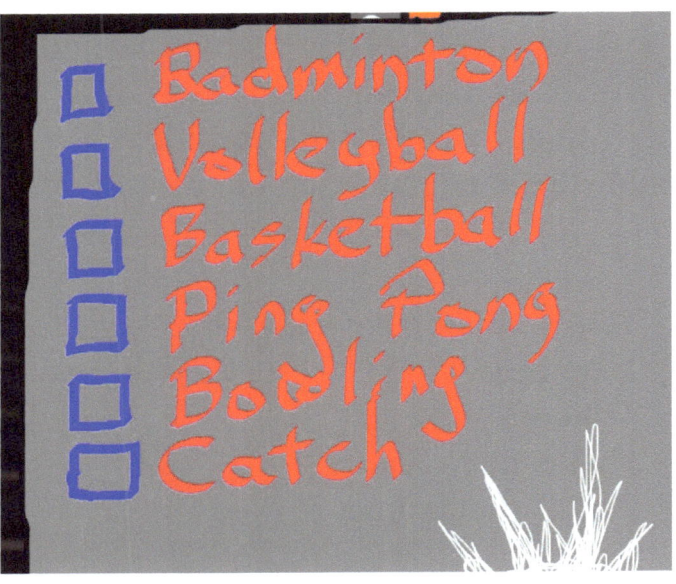

Great. Now, let's make a list of possible activities, and that should be enough to get started: Badminton, Volleyball, Basketball, Ping Pong, Bowling, Baseball, Catch, HORSE, Hide-and-Seek, Roller Skating, Roller Blading, Skiing, Biking, Rope Jumping, Jumping Jacks, Running, Walking, Skipping, Hopping, Balancing, Racing, Dancing, Marching, Playing Frisbee, Flying a Kite, Yard work…,

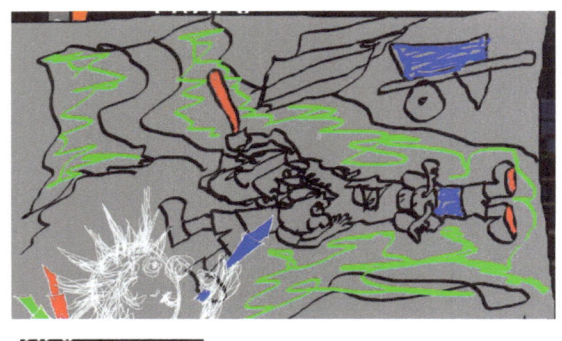

What? You don't think yard work should be in there? Yard work is a great activity. You may not like doing it, but it's a great work out.

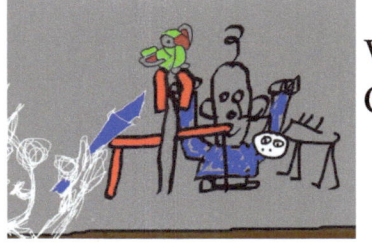

What about Musical Chairs? Yes.

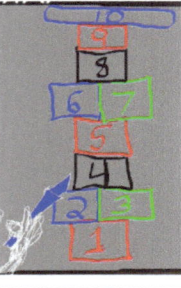

Hopscotch? Absolutely.

Anything that gets you moving , either in a small way, like ping pong, or in a big way, like basketball or roller skating. It's all about movement. Movement is good. Movement is what you need to do.

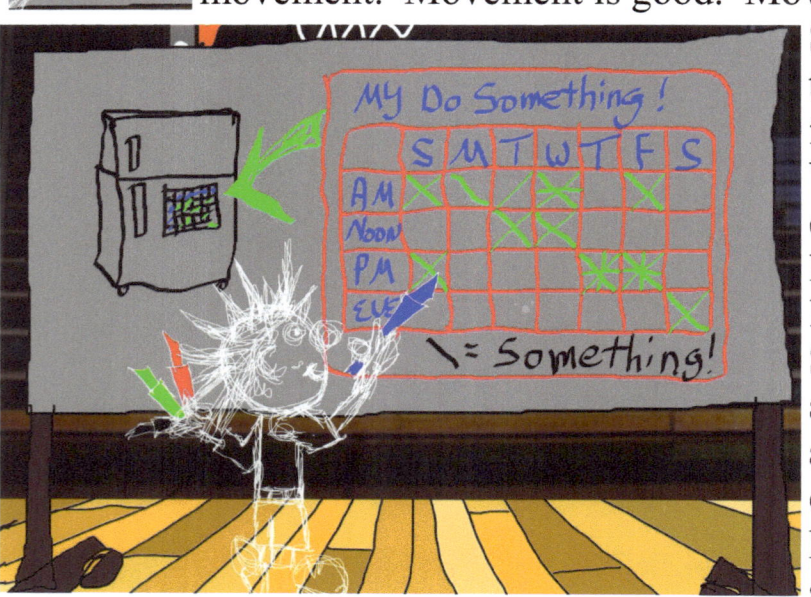

So, in making a plan, you eventually will want a schedule that fits your normal day.
When should you do your exercising?
It doesn't matter. Some people like to do things in the morning. Some people like to do things at noon. For some people, the afternoon is best. It all depends on the individual.
I like to change things around, so that I'm not always doing the same thing at the same time every day. You need your own schedule.

The most important thing to keep in mind is make a plan that you use. If you don't use the plan, change it.

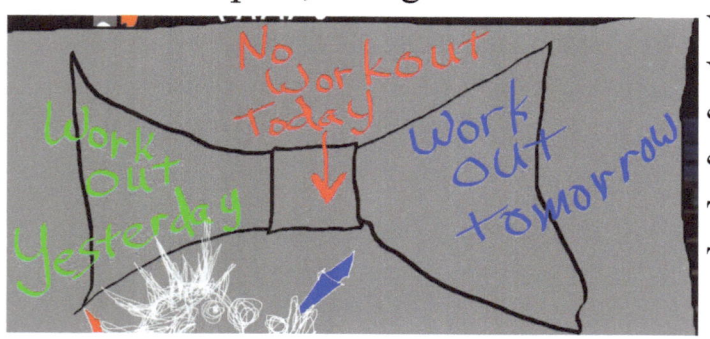

Yes?
You want to make a plan that says "Tomorrow" and "Yesterday" but not "Today"?
That is not a plan.
That is pretending.

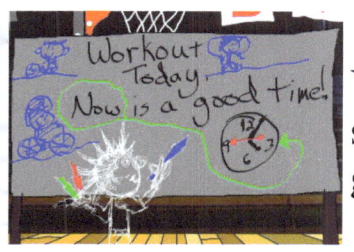

Your plan should say "Today" and it should also say "Now" so it reminds you to do something, today, and right now is a great time.

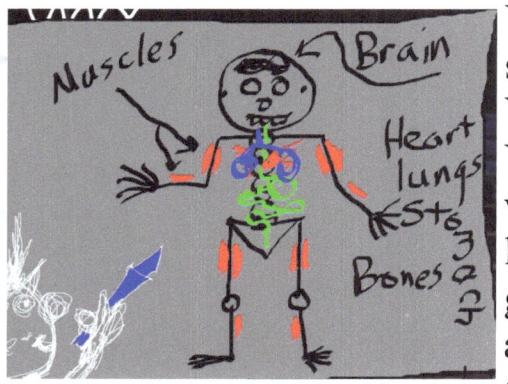

Your body is a lot like a machine: It has bones for structure. It has muscles to move things around. You need fuel (food) and oxygen to make it run. Your muscles get stronger with use and weaker with just sitting around. Strong muscles help you live better. A healthy diet makes for proper growth, including bones, teeth, skin, body tissues, and when you need to replace old, worn out cells (which is every day of your life.) Even your eyes need fuel (to see.) Your ears need fuel to hear. Your brain, especially, needs fuel, to think.

You also need to look at your body as a system: You have a brain, and a heart, lungs, a mouth, a stomach, intestines, muscles, blood in a blood stream, lots and lots of things all working together, like a team, all inside your skin (and even your skin is part of the team.)

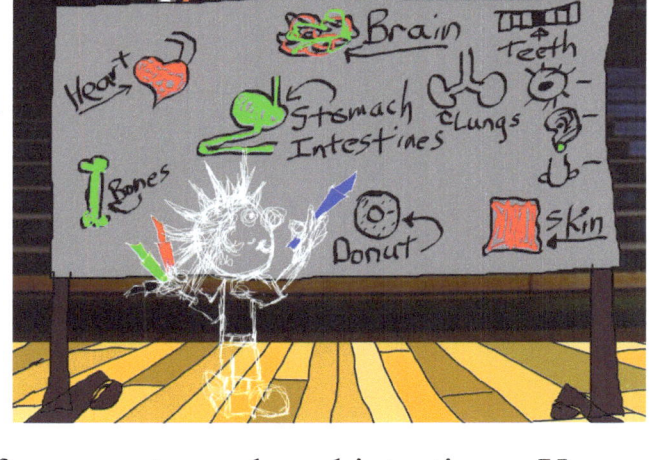

Your brain cannot eat, but it needs food. Your mouth has to do the eating. Your hands, and sometimes your legs and feet, help.

Your lungs cannot digest food; That's for your stomach and intestines. Your toes cannot get their own oxygen and nutrients. The blood stream and blood cells do that.

Your legs cannot move unless your brain tells them what to do by sending a message through your nerves.

To stay healthy, your body needs to fight diseases and heal injuries.

All of these things, combined, make up your body's ability to be/stay alive, and you have to do things with that "system" idea in mind to be, and stay, as

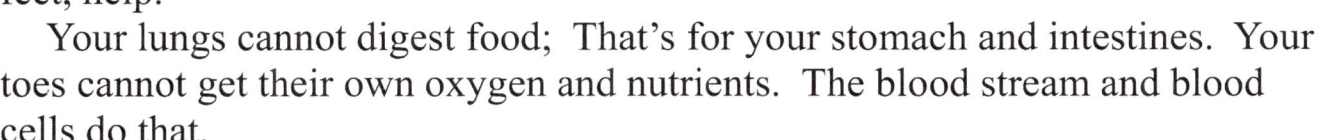

healthy as you can.

Once you have a plan, keep track of your progress.

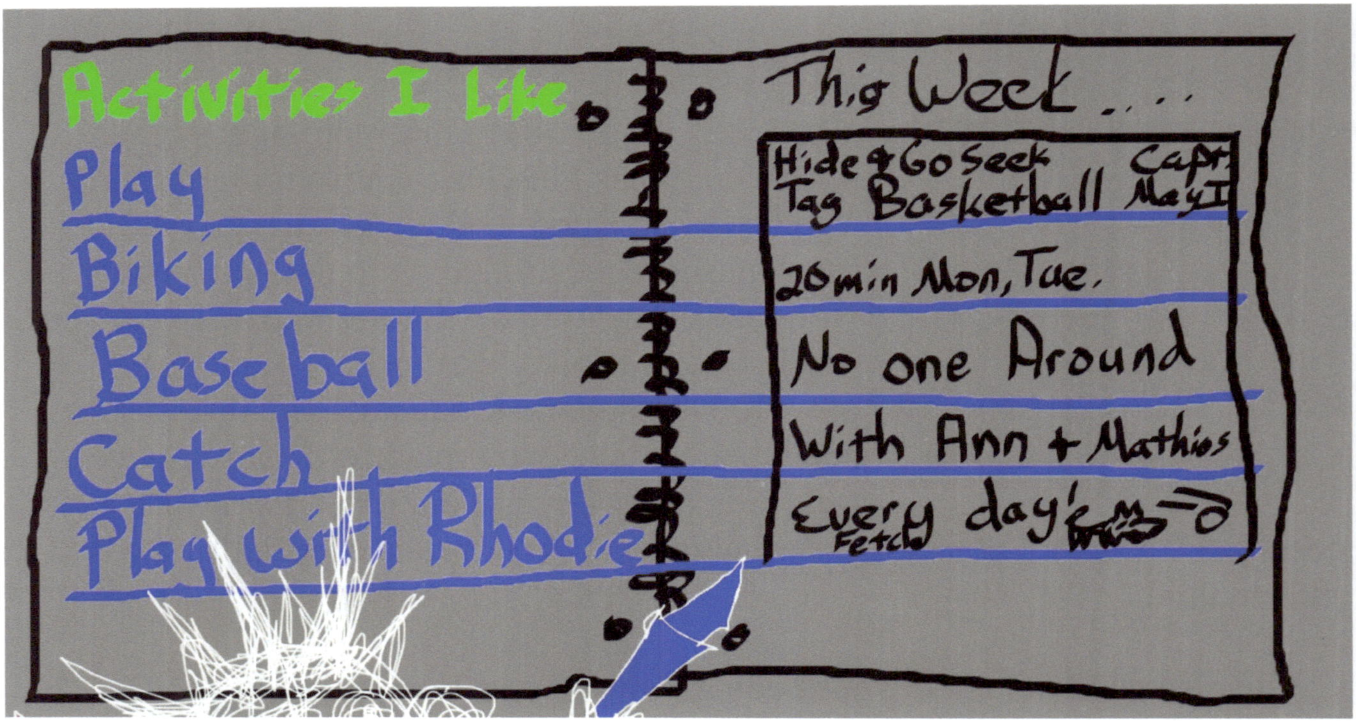

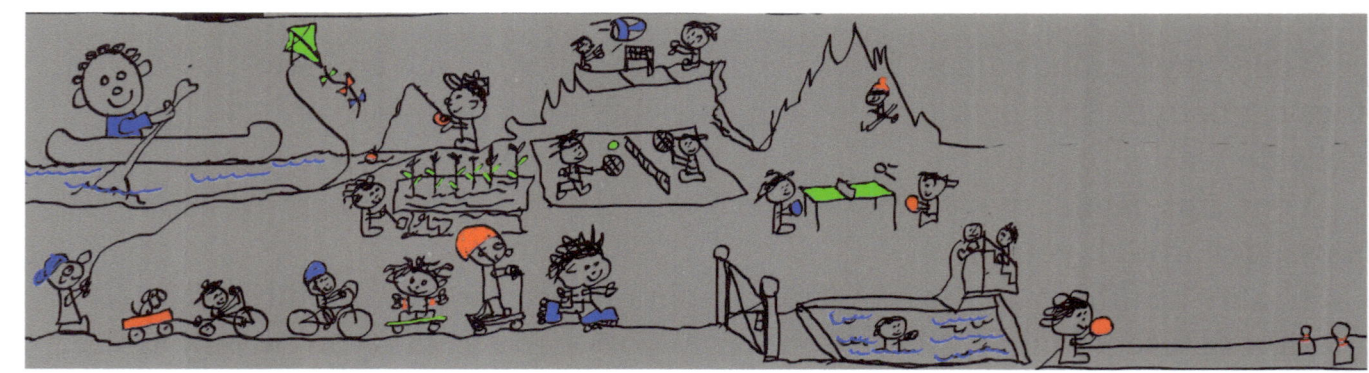

Activities I Like. | **This Week . . . .**

Play — Hide & Go Seek, Tag Basketball, Capt. May I

Biking — 20 min Mon, Tue.

Baseball — No one Around

Catch — With Ann + Mathios

Play with Rhodie — Every day! Fetch

Make a chart, or a journal, or both. Why journal? Well, it's all about thinking: Training your brain. You have to train your brain, and it's your brain that has to tell itself to be trained, and sometimes that gets confusing. Make a schedule, keep track with a chart, and write in a journal. All of those things help you to keep your body, and brain, is tip-top health.

So, well, there you have it. Now all you need to do is "Do Something!"

Keeping Record

	Large Motor	Hand-eye	Endurance	Flexibility	Brain
Sun	☐ Biking	☐ Frisbee	☐ Biking	☐ Bend	☐ Journal
Mon	☐ Roller blady	☐ Catch	☐ Jogging	☐ Stretch	☐ Plan
Tue	☐ Soccer	☐ Ping Pong	☐ Hockey	☐ TouchToes	☐ Dance
Wed	☐ Walk dog	☐ Basketball	☐ Skiing	☐ Gymnastics	☐ Teams
Thu	☐ Walk dog	☐ Bowling	☐ Swimming	☐ Ballet	☐ Be Creative
Fri	☐ Rope Skip	☐ Volleyball	☐ Tennis	☐ Rock Wall	☐ Write
Sat	☐ Swimming	☐ Football	☐ Horse Riding	☐ Diving	☐ Draw

Like make up a new game

Weekly Records

Ht		Goals:	Notes:
Wt			
Heart			
Exercise Log: Min			

What did I eat

	Sun	Mon	Tue	Wed	Thu	Fri	Sat
Fruits							
Veggies							
Proteins							
Fats							
Carbos							
Whole Grain							
Milk/Cheese							
Fats							

Excuses: Don't forget to keep track of your "excuses" for not doing. Be Creative! (and then don't use them.)

19

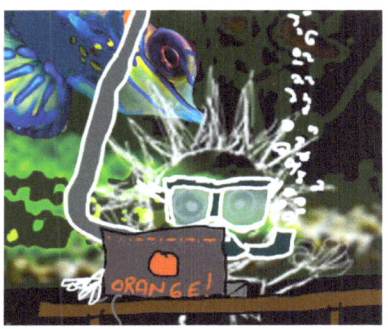

CCoQ&A

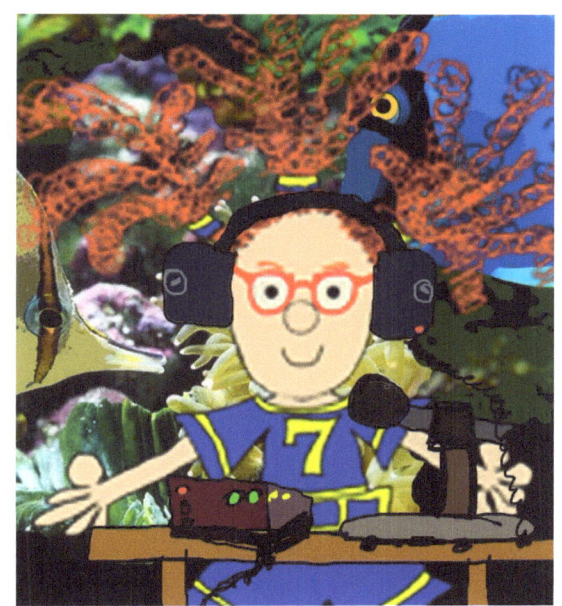

Howdy, everyone. My name is Angie Ropp, this is my best friend, "Oh, Snap!". Goulasche Press is behind the camera and you're watching "Do Something!" The show where we say, "Do something!" and then we show you something to do.

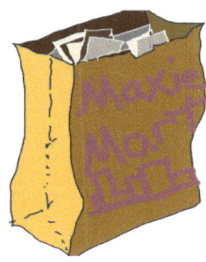

Our show, today, is what we call our "Combination Collection of Questions and Answers." We have a grocery sack full of cards and letters, sent in by people from around the neighborhood, and the nation, and even from around the world, asking questions about exercise and health: How to start, get smarter and be fit.

We're also online. "Oh, Snap!" has her laptop fired up and ready to go, so, if you're near the internet, send us an email.

We'll answer as many as we can. If we don't get to your question, we'll still send you a reply, later on this week (after I've finished with my homework, of course) and, as always, Goulasche will post them online.

Now, "Oh, Snap!" why don't you take a card from the bag and read it.

Thank you. The first card is from "Oh, Snap!" and she wants to know…,

"Oh, Snap!" what are you doing?

Just read the question? Okay.

"Oh, Snap!" would like to know: "Where are we broadcasting from?"

Well, that's a very good question. Goulasche, where are we broadcasting from, today?

Oops? What? We're broadcasting from Oops? Where's Oops?

Oh, just a minute…

(Technical Difficulties.)

While Goulasche is making a few adjustments, I'd like to say that...

Okay, then.

Is everything ready?

Oh, that's cool. Wow!

We are broadcasting, live, from a hot air balloon, flying, where? The Grand Canyon.

Sweet. Thank you, Goulasche, for that technical wizardry.

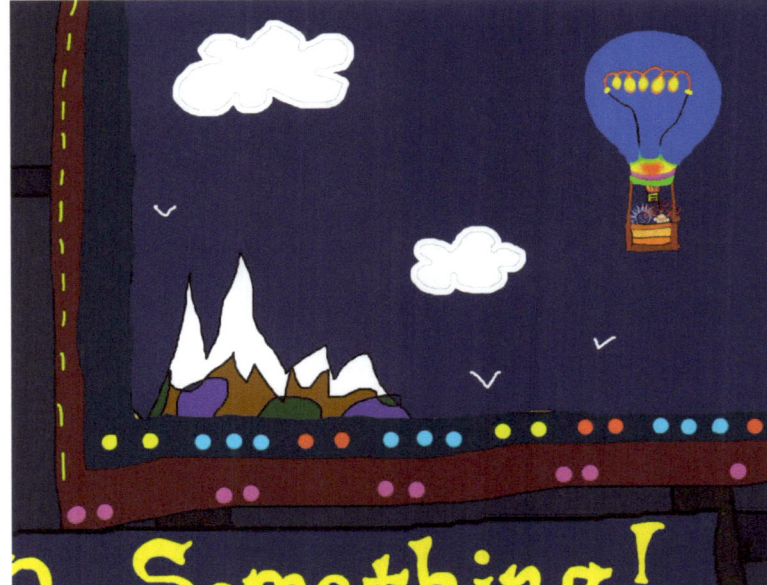

Our first card is from Dave and Bupie in Muncie, Indiana.

Dear Angie Ropp and "Oh, Snap!" "Is walking the dog exercise?"

Yes, it is. Walking the dog is great exercise, for both you and your dog. You'd be amazed at how much a dog likes to go out for a walk, and how healthy it is.

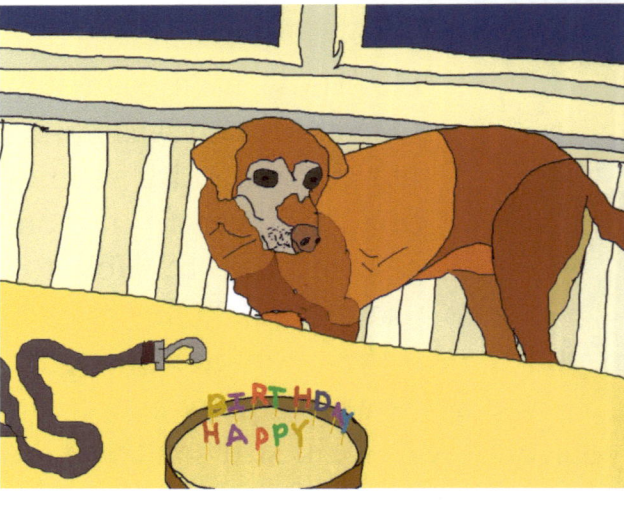

"Oh, Snap!" what's so funny?

"Walk the Dog" is also a dance? Oh, right. That is funny.

And so is "Grocery Shopping"? Yes, it is. Make sure you check your list.

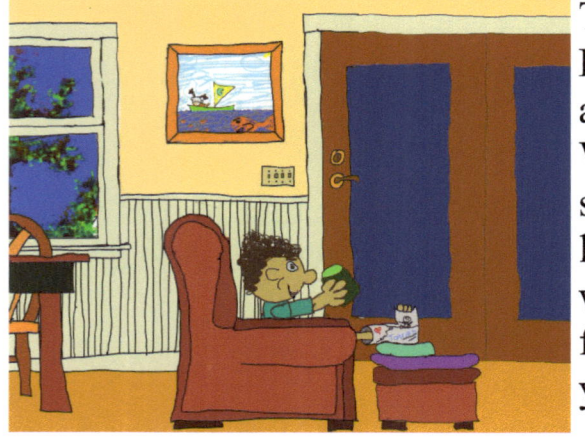

The next card is from Shannon in Las Vegas. Dear Angie and "Oh, Snap!" "I hurt my foot and can't go outside. What can I do?" Wow, that's not nice being injured. You can still do some arm exercises while sitting, like lifting weights. If you don't have any weights, use cans of fruit or a milk carton filled with water. Even a little lifting, while you're foot is healing, will be good for you.

22

Next card is from Sandy and Teri in Maryland.

Dear AR and OS. We like to go bowling, but we don't have a bowling alley in town. Any ideas?

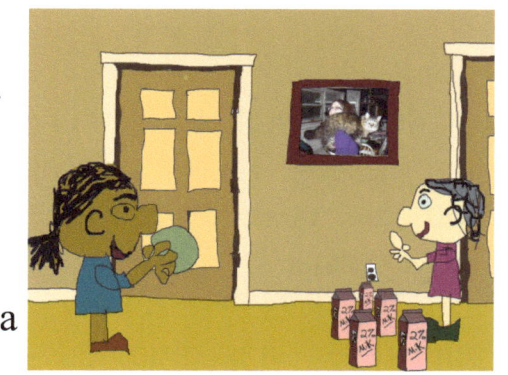

Yes. Get some empty cartons (like those little milk cartons from school.) Rinse them out and let them dry. They make excellent bowling pins. Use a softball or a tennis ball to roll at them.

No throwing inside the house, and please ask for permission and don't try to break anything.

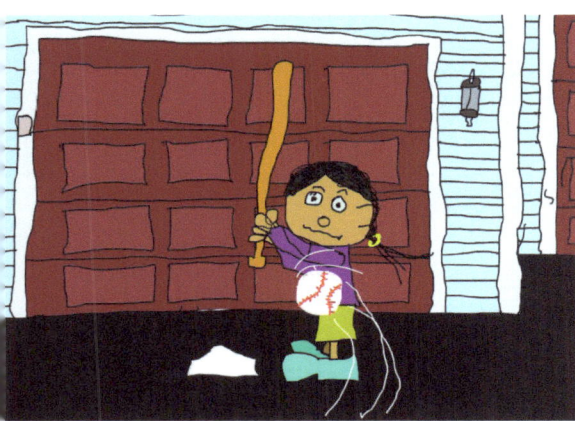

Next card…, Oh, it's an email, from Florida: Dear Angie and "Oh, Snap!" We like to play baseball, but we're the only kids in the neighborhood. What can we do? Signed Karen and Dennis. (PS. I'm younger and taller. K.)

Well, playing baseball with two people can be a problem, unless you have a plastic bat and a whiffle ball.

One person pitches. The other one hits. Fly balls caught are outs. Strike outs are outs. Balls hit are counted as singles, doubles, triples or home runs, depending upon where they land. Grounders straight to the pitcher are outs.

Make up your own teams and names. Keep track of who's up, who's on base and how many outs.

When you get three outs, switch.

Play a set number of innings; 4 or 5 usually work well.

Here's another email: This one is from Iris in Magdeburg, Germany.

"Ich habe einen Schrittzähler. Was kann ich damit machen?"

Well, "Oh, Snap!" Time to do a little online translating.

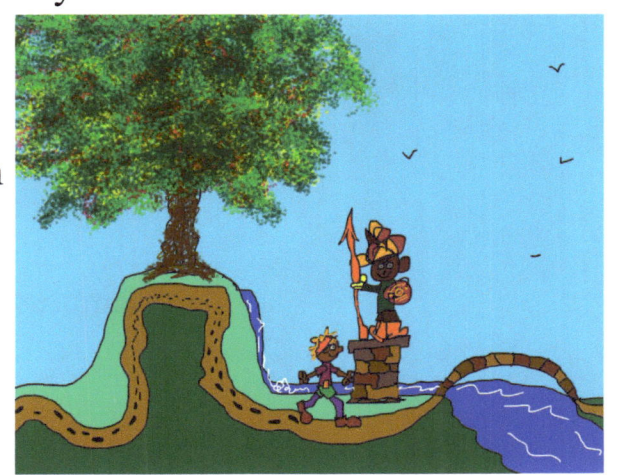

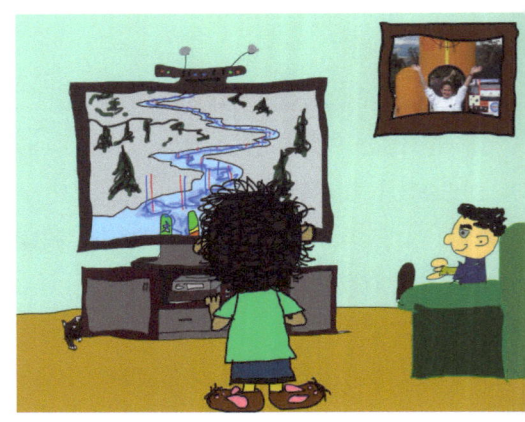

While "Oh, Snap!" is translating, I'll read a text message I received from Taino: We have a computer connected to the television. Is that really exercise?

Yes, it is. Especially if you play for an extended period of time, like 15-20 minutes, without stopping. You'll have a great workout, and you'll have fun, too. Watch out for tree branches and falling off cliffs.

Now, for our Lightning Round.
I'll read a question and answer it as quickly as I can.
Let's see how many we can do in 1 minute:

Ready? Set! Read...

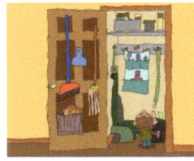

Tony in Topeka. Housework: Is that exercise?
Yes. Get a broom. Take out the garbage. Hang up your coat.

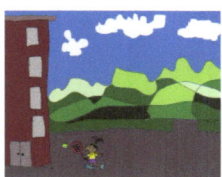

Pat in San Fransisco: I like tennis, but sometimes nobody's around? What can I do?
Use the side of a building, like at school, in the parking lot, if it's safe and permitted.

This next person didn't sign a name: Sometimes I don't feel like working out.. I just feel like sitting. Is that okay?

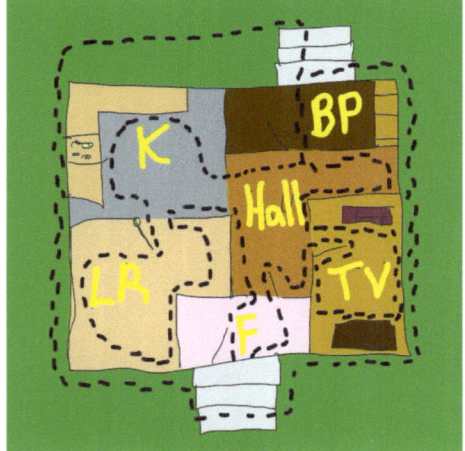

Your feelings are one thing. Your exercising is another. "Do Something!" everyday. The easiest way to overcome this is to do something simple, like go for a short walk, around the house. Make 2 laps. Maybe three. Count the steps. Make a circuit. Walk 10 "Laps". Do the math. Before you know it, 15 minutes have gone by, you have exercised a nice amount, and, well, that's one way to start. Repeat.

Yes, "Oh, Snap!" You have a little story with repeat? Okay, let's hear it"

Pete and Repeat were walking across a bridge. Pete fell off. Who was left?

Repeat.

Pete and Repeat were walking across a bridge. Pete fell off. Who was left?

Repeat.

Pete and Repeat…

Oh, that is so not funny.

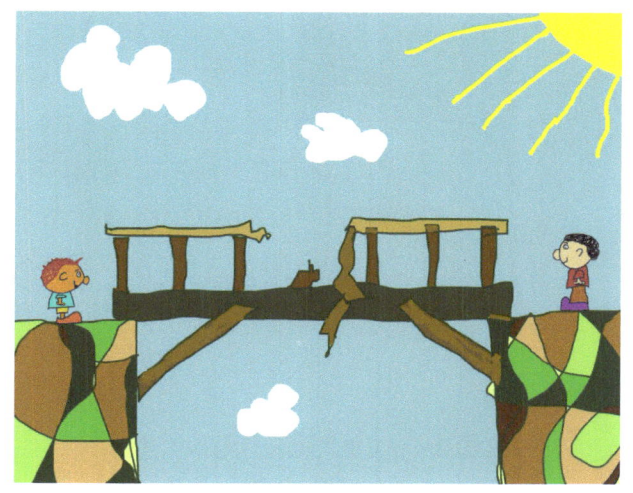

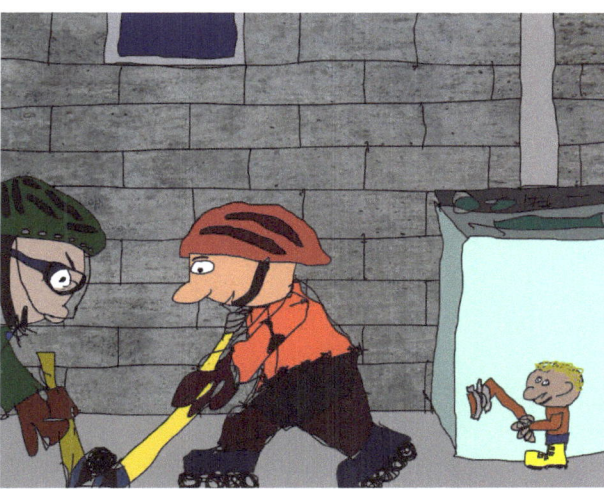

Everett from Cordova: My little brother is a pest and bothers me when I want to do something? How can I keep him away? Well, A.) Have him join in for a while. B.) Take turns. C.) Have him play for a bit and then sit. D.) Make a time with him and then make another time when he stays away. (Everyone wants to be included.)

This is from a group in Indiana: One kid always hogs the ball. When we complain, he leaves (with the ball!) What can we do?

Well, talk. Tell him how you feel. Make up some rules that everyone agrees to. Maybe he isn't very good at it and doesn't want anyone to know.

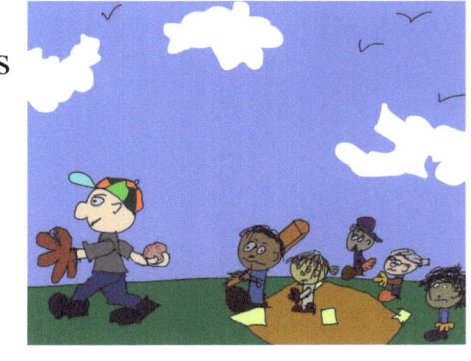

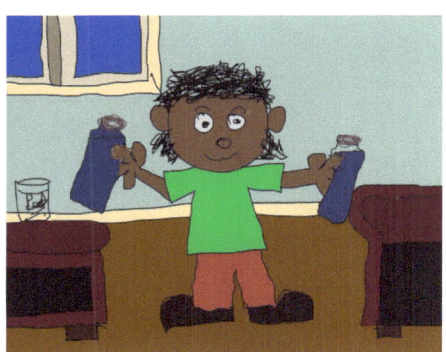

Eunice from St. Joseph: I want to life weights, but don't have any and can't afford any? Cans of fruit or vegetables work nicely. Books in a bag or backpack. Empty milk and juice jugs filled with water. A bag of flour (or sugar.) An iron skillet is very heavy. A kitty litter bucket. Bag of dog food.

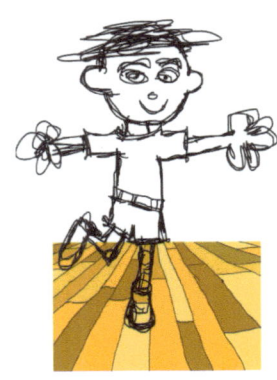

John From Salt Lake City: How can I practice my balancing without a balance beam?
Pick one floor board in the house and walk along that line down the hall and back. Don't step off the line. Wall-walking (outside on short walls, be safe.) Stand on one foot with your eyes closed: Touch your nose with your pointer finger (once with each hand.)

Roxanne from Des Moines: I want to play basketball, but it's too cold outside?
Get the newspaper out of the recycle bin. Take one page at a time, make a nice tight ball, and throw it back into the bin, for that last-second game winner.

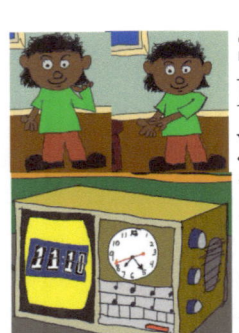

Stanley from St. Paul: How do I measure my heart rate?
Put your finger (not your thumb) on your wrist, or on the side of your head, or on the side of your neck. Find your pulse. (It's there, so keep trying.)
When you find it, count the beats while watching a clock with a second hand. Count for 1 minute. Or count for 30 seconds and multiply by 2, or count for 10 seconds and multiply by 6. That is how many times your heart beats in a minute.

Jimmy in Lexington: Some people call me Chubs. Why? I'm not chubby, but everyone makes fun of me. How much should I weigh? How do I know if I'm overweight?
Wow! Some people are not nice and they need to learn to be friendly. You can't make people be nice, but you can remind them.
As for your weight, it depends upon your age and your height. Ask your doctor, or your school nurse, or your gym teacher. It's important to be at a proper weight (not too heavy, not too light.)
If you weigh more than you should, you

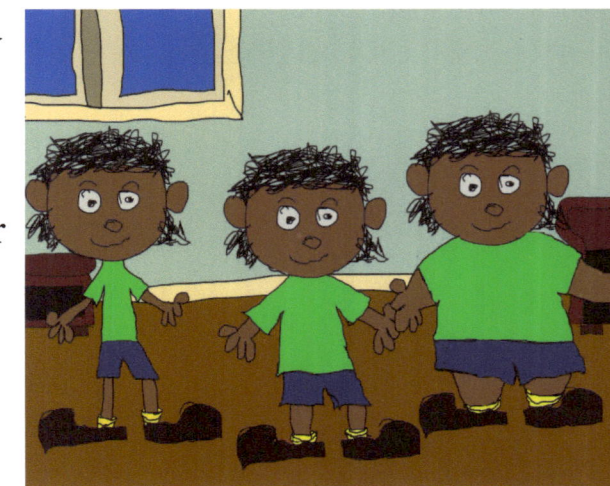

26

need a plan to lose some weight that has both diet (what you eat) and exercise goals. You can't change your weight overnight. Make a Plan. Gee, like a chart, with goals, and then a program to meet those goals, with daily progress. Don't pretend. Do something.

Having a proper weight while you are growing will help you have a proper weight after you are grown.

Brian in New London: How can I exercise inside when I'm not supposed to run around the house?

Wow: That sometimes is difficult.

What? You'll demonstrate. Okay.

"Oh, Snap!" will demonstrate exercises, at home, that don't involve running around and breaking things.

You call them your "Daily Dozen?" Okay, go.

1. Lunges.
2. Toe raises.
3. High knee walks.
4. Walk up/down the stairs ten times.
5. Do squats every time there's a food commercial on TV - keep squatting until the commercial ends.
6. Wall-sits: hold while singing the ABCs forwards and backwards.
7. Push ups: Ten times.
8. Crunches: Ten times.
9. Mountain Climbers: Ten times.
10. Burpies: Ten Times.
11. Toe Touchers: Ten Times.
12. Jumping Jacks: 157 times. How many? 157. No way. You can do 157 Jumping Jacks, without stopping? I can't make it past 75.

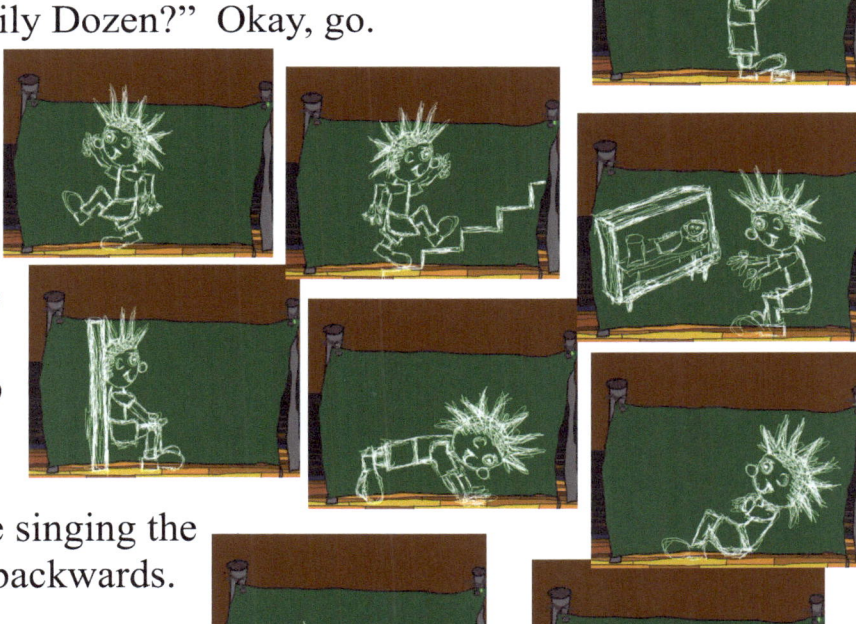

You want to show us, now?

Okay.

Ladies and Gentlemen, Boys and Girls: "Oh, Snap!" will now attempt to do 157 Jumping Jacks, without stopping.

Ready? Set! Jump...

1, 2, 3, 4, 5, 6, 7, 8, 9, 10
2, 2, 3, 4, 5, 6, 7, 8, 9, 10
3, 2, 3, 4, 5, 6, 7, 8, 9, 10
4, 2, 3, 4, 5, 6, 7, 8, 9, 10
5, 2, 3, 4, 5, 6, 7, 8, 9, 10
6, 2, 3, 4, 5, 6, 7, 8, 9, 10
7, 2, 3, 4, 5, 6, 7, 8, 9, 10
8, 2, 3, 4, 5, 6, 7, 8, 9, 10
9, 2, 3, 4, 5, 6, 7, 8, 9, 10
10, 2, 3, 4, 5, 6, 7, 8, 9, 10
11, 2, 3, 4, 5, 6, 7, 8, 9, 10
12, 2, 3, 4, 5, 6, 7, 8, 9, 10
13, 2, 3, 4, 5, 6, 7, 8, 9, 10
14, 2, 3, 4, 5, 6, 7, 8, 9, 10
15, 2, 3, 4, 5, 6, 7, 8, 9

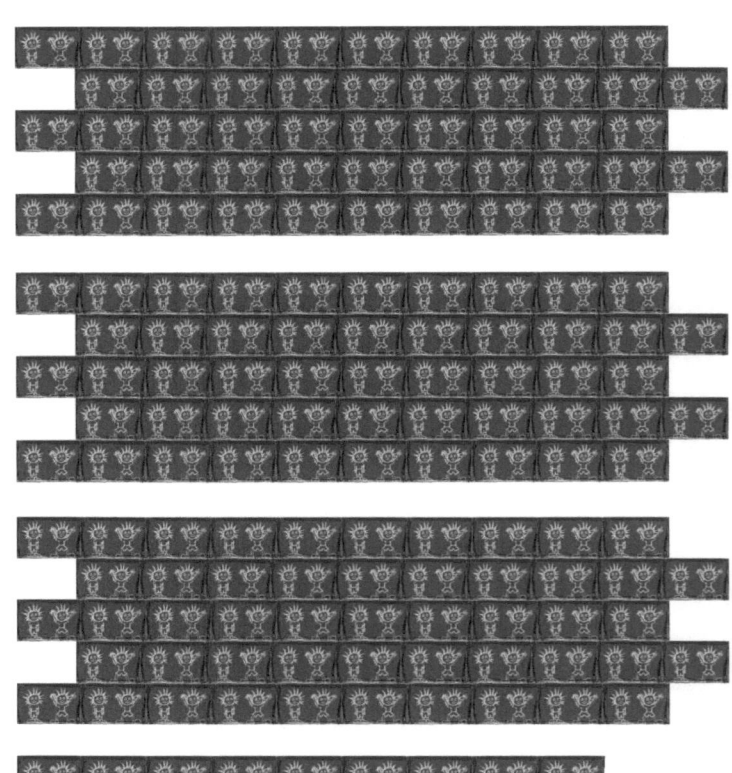

Wow! 159. That's incredible. A new record for you, too. You must be tired. I know I would be. Whew!

Well, that's going to do it for our show. We'd like to thank...,
What? Oh, right. Iris from Magdeburg.
"Ich habe einen Schrittzähler. Was kann ich damit machen?"
And that means...
"I have a pedometer. What can I do with that?"
Oh, sweet. That is one of the best things to have.
You don't know what a pedometer is?
It's a Ped-Ometer. Ped-Counter. You know: Ped - Foot. It counts your steps.

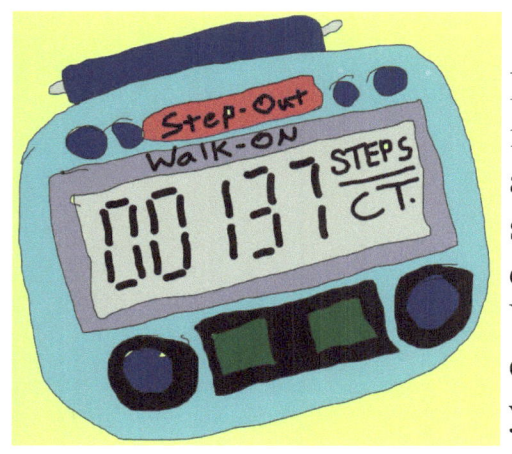

If you put in on in the morning and wear it all day, it will count how many steps you take, walking around the house, going outside, to the car or bus, shopping, school, playing sports, everything you do, counting all your steps.

Where can you get one? Any sports store, or online. You could ask for one for your birthday, if you like.

Well, that's our show. Tune in next time, for our special program called "Team Sports." It's going to be great. And remember, there is no "I" in team.

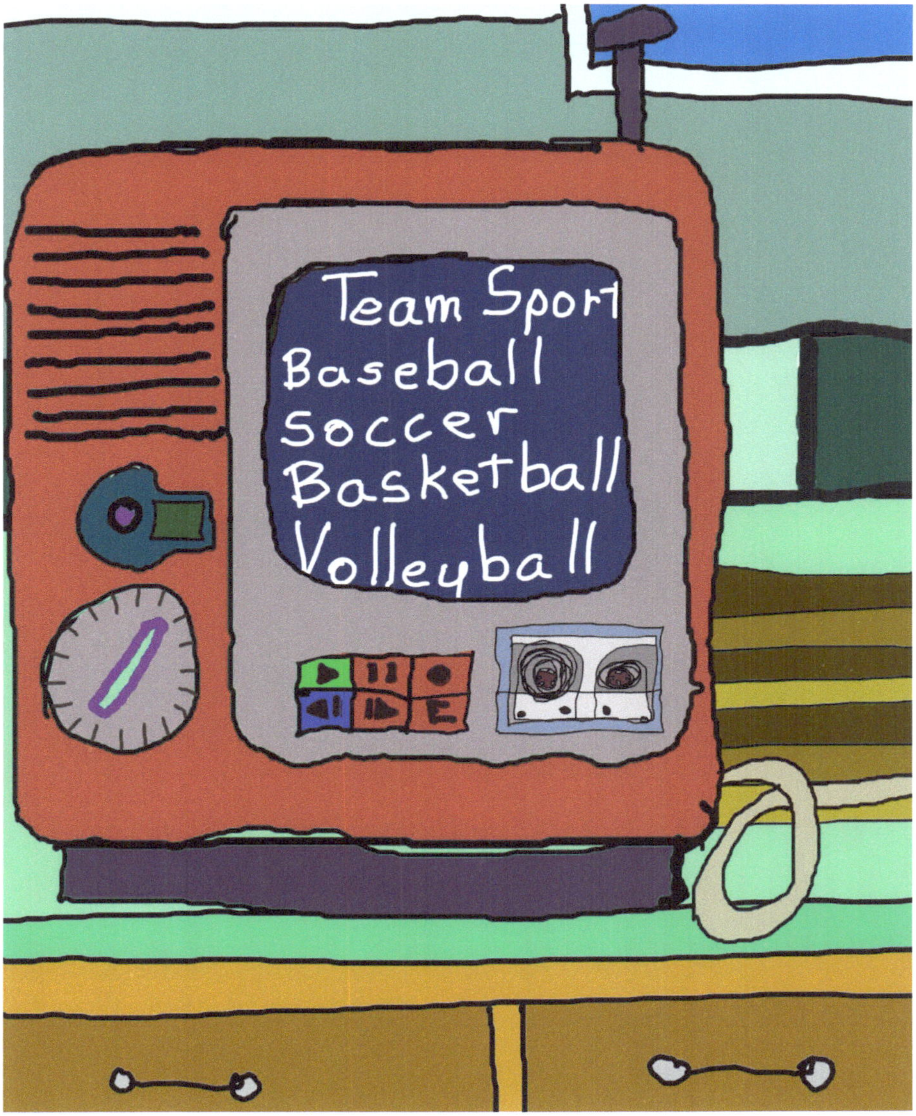

Yes, there is "ate" in TEAM,
   and "eat"
   and "at"
   and "met"
   and "am"
   and "ma"
   and "mat"
   and "met".

Bye, everybody.

(Whew! That was a great show. Thank you, Goulasche. Thank you, "Oh, Snap!" As soon as we're finished cleaning up, I think we all should go for a nice, long walk around the lake to relax and stretch out our muscles.)

"Do, Something!"